WEIGHT LOSS AFTER 60

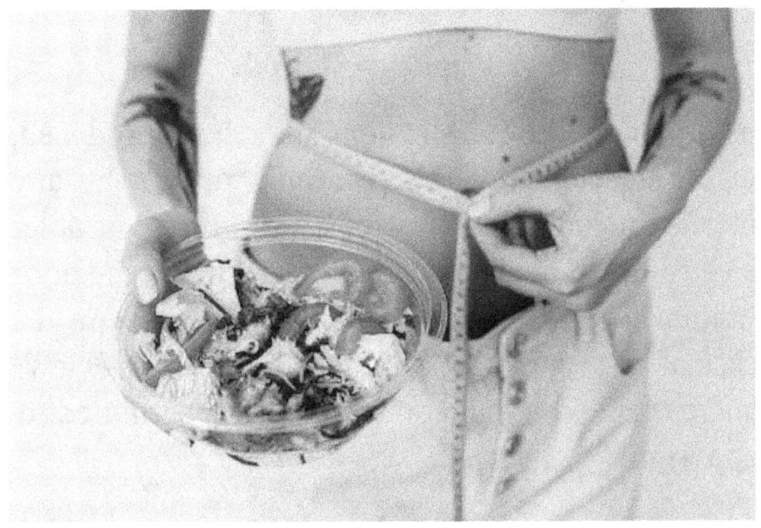

The Complete Guide and 20 Recipes for Achieving

Lasting Weight Loss for Men and Women

Wilbert M. Jensen

GAIN ACCESS TO MORE BOOKS FROM ME

TABLE OF CONTENT

INTRODUCTION

Kenny, at the age of 60, found himself at a crossroads, grappling with the weight of his past decisions as well as the physical weight that burdened his body. He set out on a transformative journey toward health and vitality, determined to rewrite his story.

Kenny adopted a healthy diet that included colorful vegetables and lean proteins while saying goodbye to sugary treats. His mornings began with energizing walks, which gradually progressed into a full-fledged exercise regimen tailored to his abilities.

Kenny discovered newfound energy and a zest for life as the pounds melted away. Small victories, such as fitting into old jeans and climbing stairs with ease, encouraged him to realize that one's age does not have to dictate one's well-being. Kenny's perseverance inspired those around him, demonstrating that it's never too late to prioritize health. Kenny discovered a renewed sense of self and a vibrant chapter in the story of his golden years by losing weight.

DELICIOUS WEIGHT LOSS AFTER 60 RECIPES

Grilled Salmon with Lemon and Dill:

Salmon fillet

Lemon

Fresh dill

Olive oil

Salt and pepper to taste

Preparation: Marinate salmon with olive oil, lemon juice, dill, salt, and pepper. Grill until cooked through.

Vegetable Stir-Fry:

Mixed vegetables (broccoli, bell peppers, carrots)

Olive oil

Garlic

Ginger

Low-sodium soy sauce

Preparation: Sauté garlic and ginger in olive oil. Add vegetables and stir-fry until tender. Finish with soy sauce.

Quinoa Salad with Veggies:

Quinoa

Cucumber

Cherry tomatoes

Red onion

Olive oil and balsamic vinegar

Fresh basil

Preparation: Cook quinoa, mix with chopped vegetables, and dress with olive oil, balsamic vinegar, and fresh basil.

Chicken and Vegetable Skewers:

Chicken breast

Bell peppers

Zucchini

Olive oil

Garlic powder

Paprika

Preparation: Cut chicken and vegetables into chunks. Skewer and brush with olive oil, garlic powder, and paprika. Grill until chicken is cooked.

Sweet Potato and Kale Hash:

Sweet potatoes

Kale

Onion

Olive oil

Paprika

Salt and pepper

Preparation: Sauté diced sweet potatoes, kale, and onions in olive oil. Season with paprika, salt, and pepper.

Mango and Avocado Salad:

Romaine lettuce

Mango

Avocado

Red onion

Lime juice

Olive oil

Preparation: Toss lettuce, mango, avocado, and red onion. Dress with lime juice and olive oil.

Baked Cod with Herbs:

Cod fillet

Fresh herbs (parsley, thyme)

Lemon

Olive oil

Garlic

Preparation: Coat cod with olive oil, herbs, lemon juice, and minced garlic. Bake until fish flakes easily.

Chickpea and Spinach Curry:

Chickpeas

Spinach

Tomato

Onion

Garlic

Curry spices

Preparation: Sauté onion and garlic, add chickpeas, tomatoes, spinach, and curry spices. Simmer until flavors meld.

Turkey and Vegetable Soup:

Ground turkey

Carrots

Celery

Onion

Low-sodium broth

Thyme

Preparation: Brown turkey, sauté vegetables, add broth and thyme. Simmer until vegetables are tender.

Eggplant and Tomato Bake:

Eggplant

Tomato

Mozzarella cheese

Basil

Olive oil

Garlic

Preparation: Layer sliced eggplant, tomato, and mozzarella. Drizzle with olive oil, sprinkle with garlic and basil. Bake until bubbly.

Lentil and Vegetable Stew:

Lentils

Carrots

Potatoes

Onion

Garlic

Low-sodium broth

Preparation: Sauté onion and garlic, add lentils, carrots, potatoes, and broth. Simmer until lentils are tender.

Greek Yogurt Parfait:

Greek yogurt

Berries

Granola

Honey

Preparation: Layer Greek yogurt with berries and granola. Drizzle with honey.

Broccoli and Almond Stir-Fry:

Broccoli

Almonds

Soy sauce

Sesame oil

Ginger

Garlic

Preparation: Stir-fry broccoli, almonds, ginger, and garlic in sesame oil. Finish with soy sauce.

Turkey and Quinoa Stuffed Peppers:

Ground turkey

Quinoa

Bell peppers

Tomato sauce

Onion

Italian herbs

Preparation: Cook turkey and quinoa. Mix with tomato sauce, onion, and herbs. Stuff peppers and bake.

Cauliflower Rice Stir-Fry:

Cauliflower

Mixed vegetables

Egg

Soy sauce

Sesame oil

Preparation: Pulse cauliflower in a blender to rice-sized pieces. Stir-fry with mixed vegetables, egg, soy sauce, and sesame oil.

Spinach and Feta Omelette:

Eggs

Spinach

Feta cheese

Olive oil

Salt and pepper

Preparation: Whisk eggs, pour into a pan with spinach and feta. Cook until set. Season with salt and pepper.

Baked Chicken with Rosemary:

Chicken thighs

Rosemary

Lemon

Olive oil

Garlic

Preparation: Coat chicken with olive oil, rosemary, lemon juice, and minced garlic. Bake until golden brown.

Mushroom and Asparagus Saute:

Mushrooms

Asparagus

Olive oil

Garlic

Lemon zest

Thyme

Preparation: Sauté mushrooms and asparagus in olive oil with garlic, lemon zest, and thyme.

Cabbage and Sausage Skillet:

Cabbage

Turkey sausage

Onion

Garlic

Paprika

Salt and pepper

Preparation: Cook sausage, add cabbage, onion, garlic, paprika, salt, and pepper. Sauté until tender.

Tuna and White Bean Salad:

Canned tuna

White beans

Cherry tomatoes

Red onion

Olive oil

Lemon juice

Preparation: Mix tuna, white beans, cherry tomatoes, and red onion. Dress with olive oil and lemon juice.

MEAL PLAN

Day 1:

Breakfast: Greek yogurt with mixed berries and a sprinkle of chia seeds.

Mid-Morning Snack: Handful of almonds and a small apple.

Lunch: Grilled chicken salad with mixed greens, cherry tomatoes, cucumber, and a light vinaigrette dressing.

Afternoon Snack: Carrot and celery sticks with hummus.

Dinner: Baked salmon with steamed broccoli and quinoa.

Day 2:

Breakfast: Oatmeal with sliced banana, a teaspoon of almond butter, and a sprinkle of cinnamon.

Mid-Morning Snack: Low-fat cottage cheese with pineapple chunks.

Lunch: Lentil soup with a side of whole-grain crackers and a green salad.

Afternoon Snack: Greek yogurt with a drizzle of honey and a handful of walnuts.

Dinner: Stir-fried tofu with mixed vegetables and brown rice.

Day 3:

Breakfast: Scrambled eggs with spinach and whole-grain toast.

Mid-Morning Snack: A small orange and a handful of mixed nuts.

Lunch: Turkey and avocado whole-grain wrap with a side of raw veggies.

Afternoon Snack: Celery sticks with light cream cheese.

Dinner: Grilled chicken breast with roasted sweet potatoes and asparagus.

Day 4:

Breakfast: Smoothie with kale, banana, and low-fat milk or almond milk.

Mid-Morning Snack: Pear slices with a tablespoon of peanut butter.

Lunch: Quinoa salad with black beans, corn, tomatoes, and a lime-cilantro dressing.

Afternoon Snack: Cottage cheese with sliced peaches.

Dinner: Baked cod with quinoa and roasted Brussels sprouts.

Day 5:

Breakfast: Whole-grain waffles with Greek yogurt and mixed berries.

Mid-Morning Snack: A handful of grapes and a small handful of almonds.

Lunch: Chicken and vegetable stir-fry with brown rice.

Afternoon Snack: Yogurt with a sprinkle of granola and sliced strawberries.

Dinner: Grilled shrimp with quinoa and a side of steamed broccoli.

Day 6:

Breakfast: Cottage cheese pancakes with sliced strawberries and a drizzle of maple syrup.

Mid-Morning Snack: Plum slices and a handful of walnuts.

Lunch: Chickpea and vegetable curry with a side of cauliflower rice.

Afternoon Snack: Carrot and cucumber sticks with hummus.

Dinner: Baked chicken thighs with a side of quinoa and mixed green beans.

Day 7:

Breakfast: Egg white omelet with spinach, tomatoes, and feta cheese.

Mid-Morning Snack: Apple slices with a tablespoon of almond butter.

Lunch: Quinoa-stuffed bell peppers with a side of mixed greens.

Afternoon Snack: Greek yogurt with a drizzle of honey and a handful of walnuts.

Dinner: Grilled fish tacos with cabbage slaw and a side of black beans.

CONCLUSION

The story of weight reduction beyond 60 resonates with victory, courage, and newfound vigor in the durable fabric of life.

It represents the steadfast spirit that resists cultural standards and believes in the transforming potential of self-care. This trip is a significant reclaiming of one's narrative—a proclamation that health is not restricted by age but rather a continuous, exciting quest.

As the scales shift as the body changes, so does the spirit. Every healthy choice, every purposeful stride becomes a booming declaration of resilience and self-love.

Weight reduction after 60 is more than just a physical shift; it is a profound transition that pervades all aspects of life. It is the unwritten manifesto that says unequivocally that the best is yet to come—a glorious homage to embracing the golden years with a rejuvenated body and soul.

Happy cooking!

Contact me